X

DIAGNOSTIC PICTURE TESTS IN

Renal Disease

Graeme R.D. Catto DSc
Professor
Department of Medicine and Therapeutics
University of Aberdeen, Scotland

Paul A.J. Brown MB, ChB
Registrar and Honorary Lecturer
Department of Pathology
University of Aberdeen, Scotland

Izhar H. Khan MRCP
Research Fellow
Department of Medicine and Therapeutics
University of Aberdeen, Scotland

N1 Mosby–Wolfe

Titles published in the Diagnostic Picture Tests in... series include:

Copyright © 1994 Times Mirror International Publishers Ltd
Published in 1994 by Mosby–Wolfe; an imprint of Times Mirror International
Publishers Ltd
Printed by Grafos S.A. Arte sobre papel, Barcelona, Spain
ISBN 0 7234 1973 6

For full details of all Times Mirror International Publishers Ltd titles please write to
Times Mirror International Publishers Ltd, Lynton House, 7–12 Tavistock Square,
London WC1H 9LB, England.

A CIP catalogue record for this book is available from the British Library.

Library of Congress Cataloging-in-Publication Data has been applied for.

ACKNOWLEDGEMENTS

The following are thanked for advice, contributions and allowing their patients to be photographed.

Dr A. Bayliss, Department of Radiodiagnosis, Aberdeen Royal Infirmary; Dr R. Herriot, Department of Pathology, Aberdeen Royal Infirmary; Dr M.A. Brown, Victoria Hospital, New South Wales, Australia; Dr A. Gemmel, Department of Nuclear Medicine, Aberdeen Royal Infirmary; Mr K.P. Duguid, Department of Medical Illustration, University of Aberdeen; Dr N. Edward, Renal Unit, Aberdeen Royal Infirmary; Dr A.G. Jardine, Department of Medicine and Therapeutics, University of Aberdeen; Dr N.E.I. Langlois, Dr S Robinson, Dr M. Taylor, and Dr E.S. Gray, Department of Pathology, University of Aberdeen; Dr A.M. MacLeod, Department of Medicine and Therapeutics, University of Aberdeen; Ms S.M. Martin, Department of Medical Illustration, University of Aberdeen; Dr A.D. Ormerod, Department of Dermatology, Aberdeen Royal Infirmary, Dr J.G. Simpson, Department of Pathology, University of Aberdeen; and Dr F. Smith, Department of Nuclear Medicine, Aberdeen Royal Infirmary.

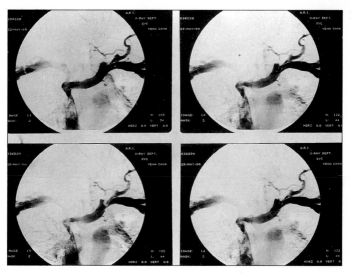

1, 2 These venograms (**1** and **2**) were performed before and after a procedure.
(a) What was the diagnosis?
(b) What procedure was performed?
(c) Which nephrological procedure may result in this complication?

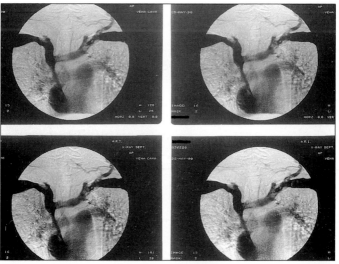

3

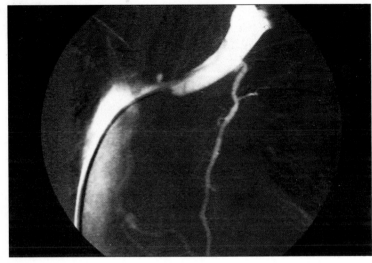

3, 4 What is shown in these venograms performed in the fistula arm of a dialysis patient?

4

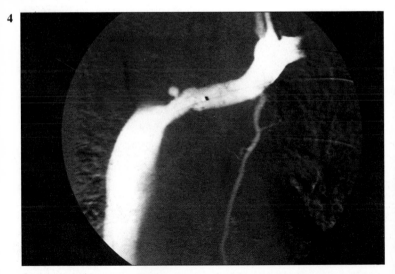

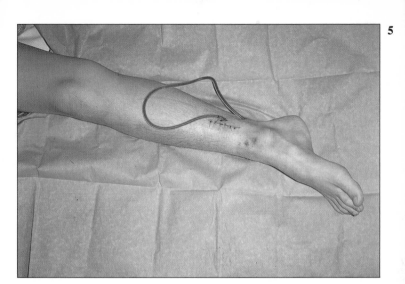

5 (a) What is shown here?
(b) What are its indications?

6 What type of vascular access is shown here?

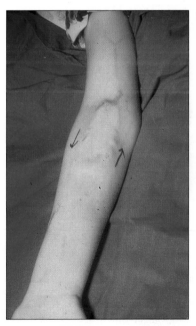

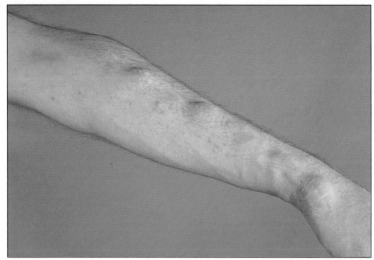

7 This is the arm of a patient who received a renal transplant one year ago. What two signs are shown?

8 What complication is seen here?

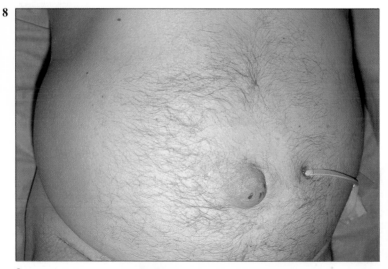

8

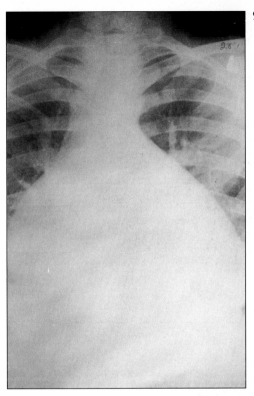

9 This chest radiograph is from a patient with uraemia.
(a) What is the diagnosis?
(b) How is it treated?
(c) What complication can occur?

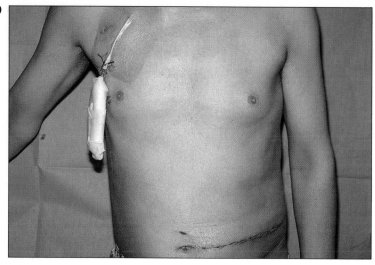

10, 11 (a) What surgical procedure has been performed?
(b) What was the diagnosis?
(c) When is such surgery indicated?

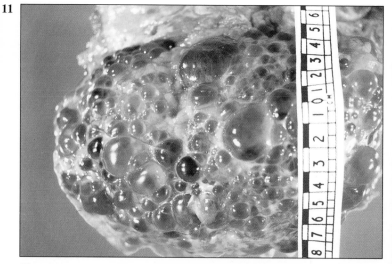

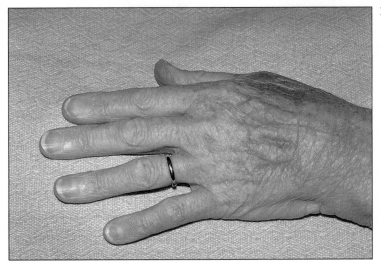

12 (a) Which pathognomonic sign is shown here?
(b) What is the diagnosis?

13

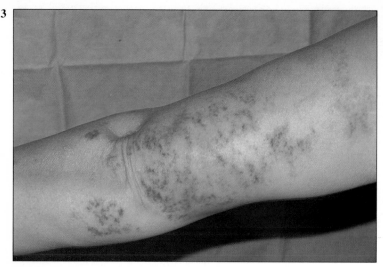

14

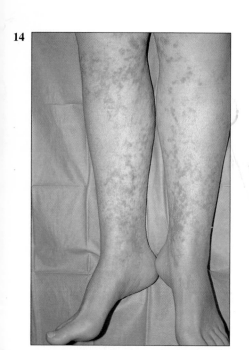

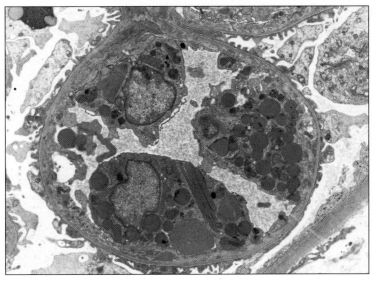

13–15 This patient presented with nephrotic syndrome.
(a) What is seen on the arm and legs?
(b) What abnormality is shown in the electron micrograph of the renal biopsy?
(c) What is the diagnosis?

16 The X-ray was taken after temporary haemodialysis. What complication has occurred?

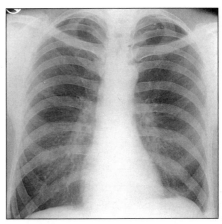

17

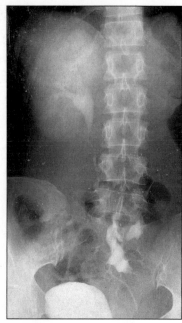

17 What is shown in this intravenous urogram?

18

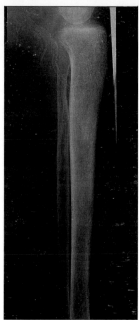

18 This plain X-ray shows a sign associated with long-standing chronic renal failure.
(a) Name the sign.
(b) Give the possible reasons.

19 (a) What investigation has been performed?
(b) What is the diagnosis?

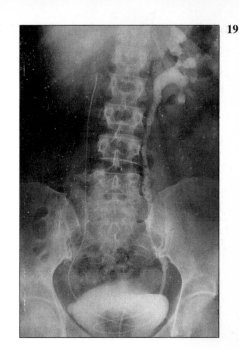

20 This patient has chronic renal failure.
(a) What are the possible causes of his renal failure?
(b) How is he being treated?

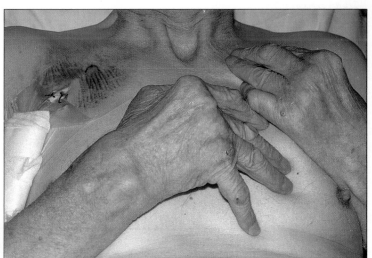

21

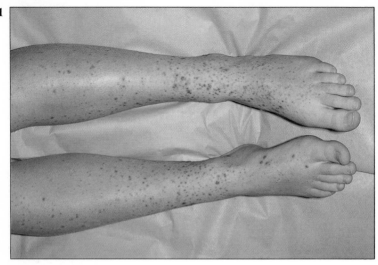

21–23 This skin lesion occurred in a ten-year-old girl.
(a) What is the diagnosis?
(b) What does the renal biopsy show?

22

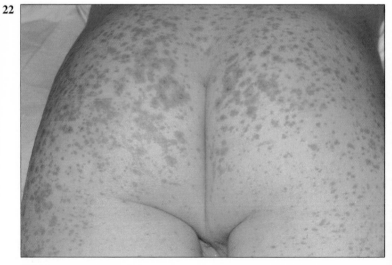

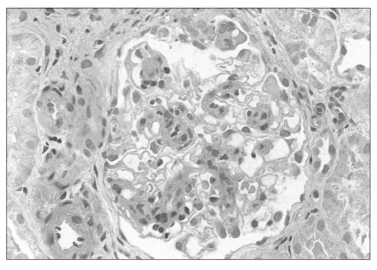

24 (a) What lesion is shown in this post-renal transplant patient?
(b) What was the likely reason?

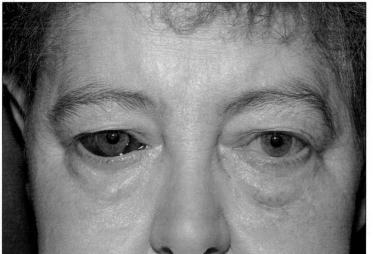

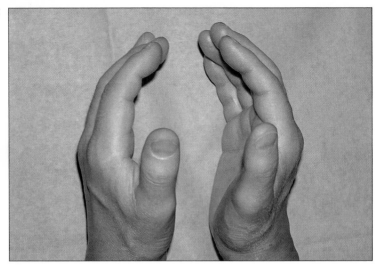

25, 26 These are the hands of a patient who has been on dialysis for 15 years. The fingers are in fixed flexion and a procedure was performed in the past.
(a) What is the cause of this deformity?
(b) What procedure was carried out?

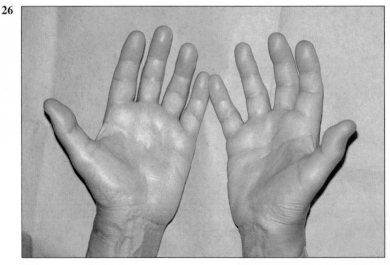

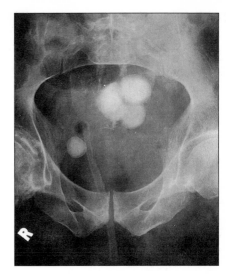

27 What is shown in this plain radiograph?

28 (a) What sign is shown?
(b) What is the cause of this condition in patients with chronic renal failure?

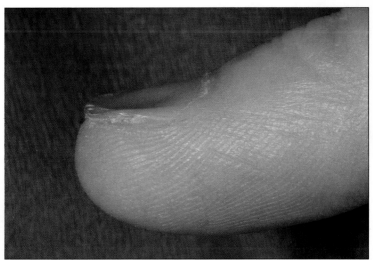

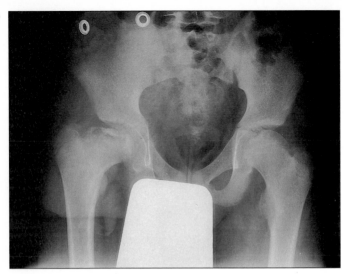

29 This is a radiograph of a child on renal replacement therapy.
(a) What abnormality is seen and why?
(b) What type of renal replacement therapy was he on?

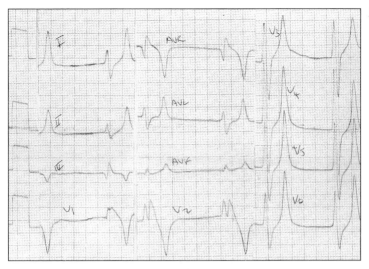

30 (a) What abnormalities are shown in this ECG?
(b) What is the diagnosis?
(c) What is the treatment of this condition?

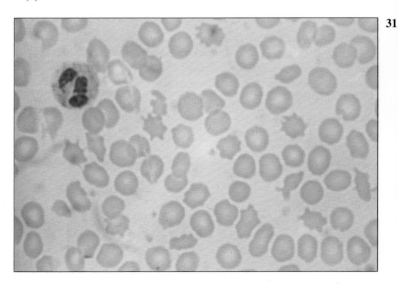

31 What abnormal features are shown in this blood film from a patient with chronic renal failure?

32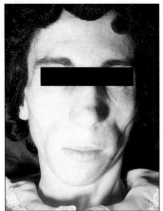

32–34 (a) What feature is illustrated in this patient's face?
(b) Name the renal biopsy lesion associated with this feature.

33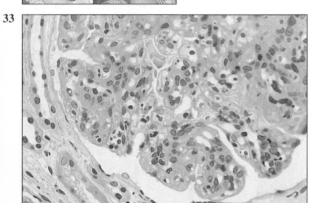

34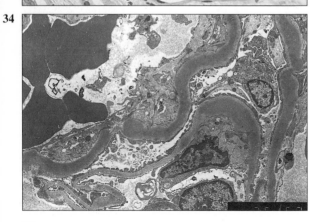

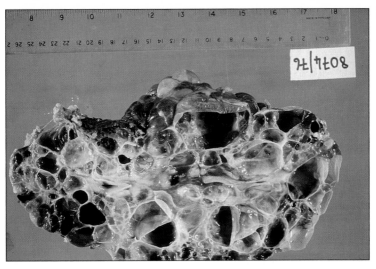

35, 36 (a) What is the diagnosis?
(b) What does microscopy of the renal lesions show?

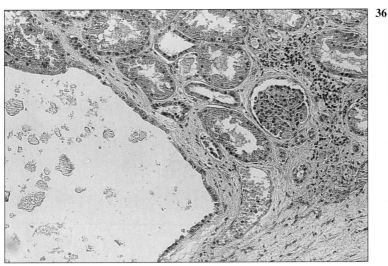

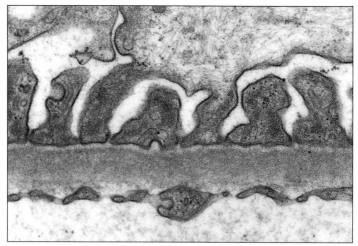

37, 38 An electron micrograph of a normal glomerular basement membrane is shown in **37**. That from a patient with familial haematuria and normal renal function is shown in **38**. What is the diagnosis?

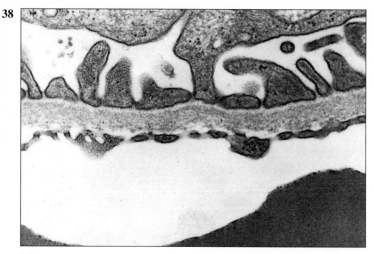

39–42 What do the gross specimen of this kidney and its histological appearance show?

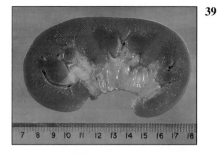

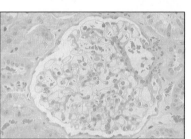

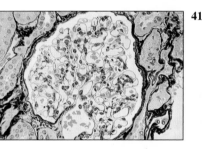

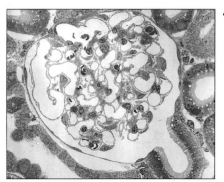

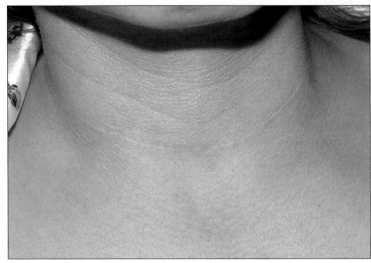

43, 44 What two signs are illustrated in this patient who is receiving maintenance haemodialysis?

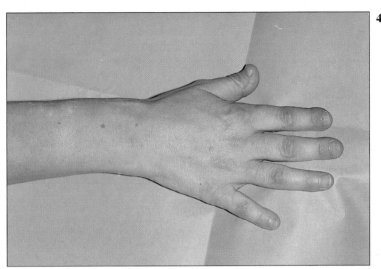

45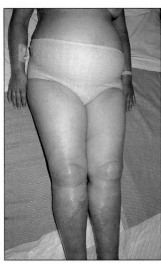

45–49 (a) Name the signs illustrated in this patient.
(b) What does the renal biopsy show?
(c) What are the clinical and pathological diagnoses?

(NB **48** is a normal electron-micrograph. **49** is from the patient.)

46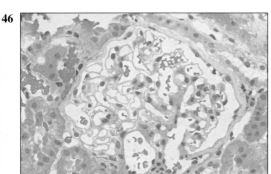

47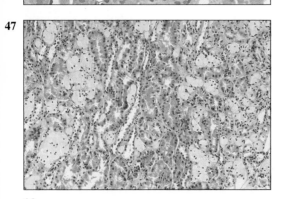

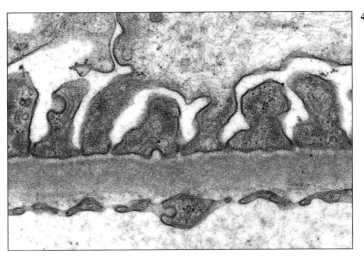

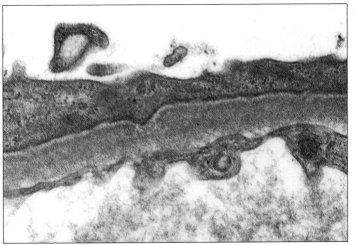

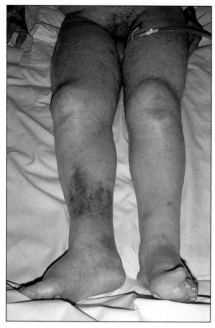

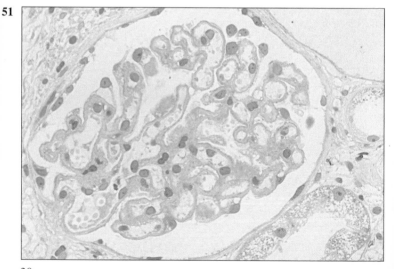

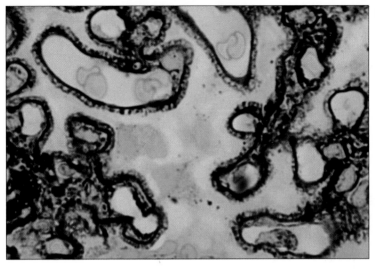

50–52 (a) Name the clinical sign shown.
(b) What does the renal biopsy show?

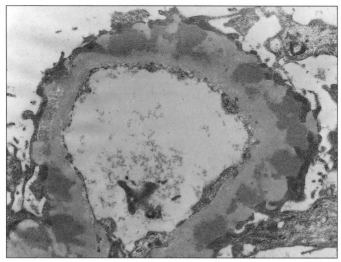

53 This electron micrograph of a renal biopsy from a patient with membranous nephropathy shows a characteristic feature within the glomerular capillary loop. Name the feature and state where it is located.

54 What abnormality is shown in this kidney from a child with a urinary tract infection?

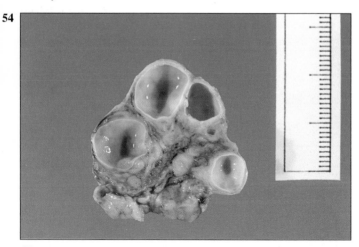

55 Name the abnormal
feature in this kidney.

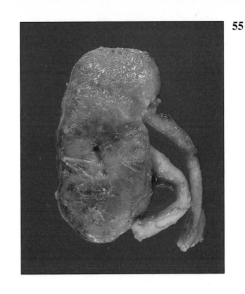

56 What complications can
occur with this congenital
anomaly?

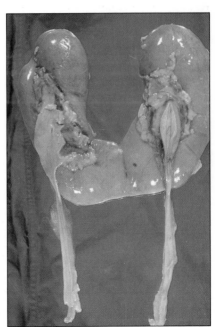

57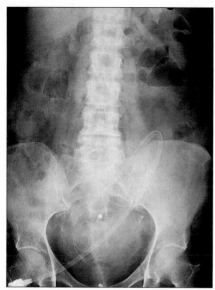

57, 58 (a) What is shown in the plain abdominal X-ray in **57**?
(b) Name the abnormality seen in the X-ray from the same patient shown in **58** following a procedure.
(c) What procedure was performed?

58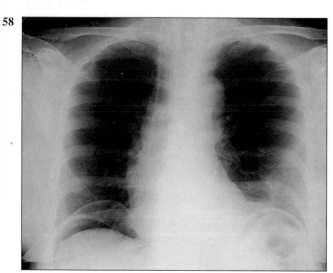

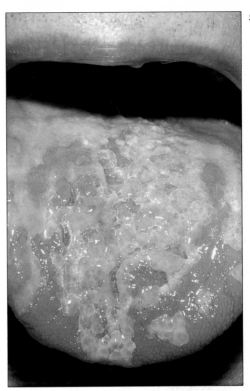

59 What is seen in this patient who has had a recent renal transplant?

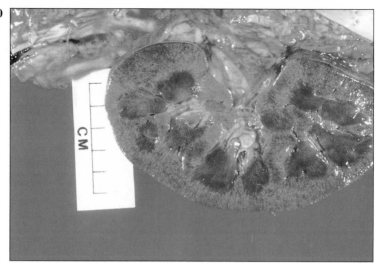

60, 61 The gross specimen and renal microscopy are from a patient who had haematuria and azotemia following a skin infection. What is the diagnosis?

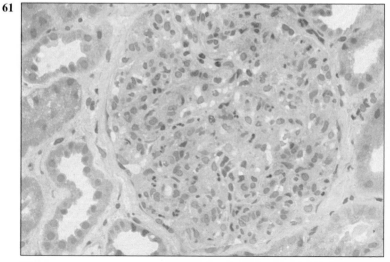

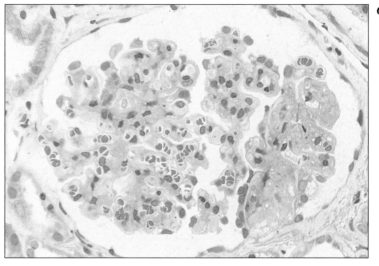

62, 63 What abnormality is seen in this glomerulus on haematoxylin–eosin and silver stain? The child had nephrotic syndrome and renal impairment.

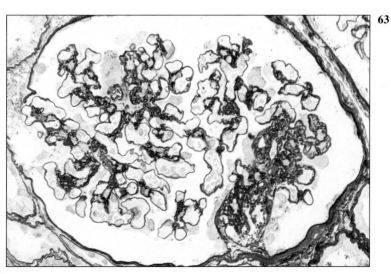

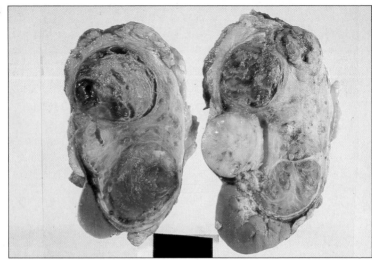

64, 65 The gross specimen of this kidney is from a four-year-old child.
(a) What is the diagnosis?
(b) What is shown on microscopy?

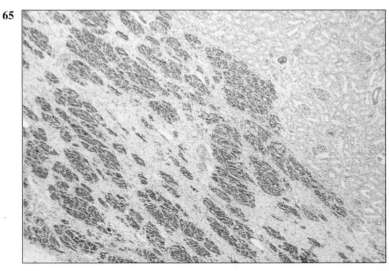

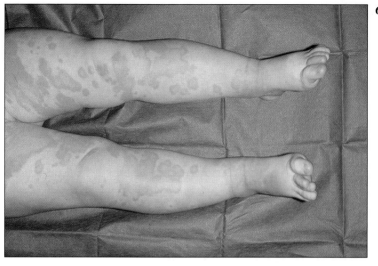

66, 67 (a) Name the lesions illustrated.
(b) What are the possible causes?

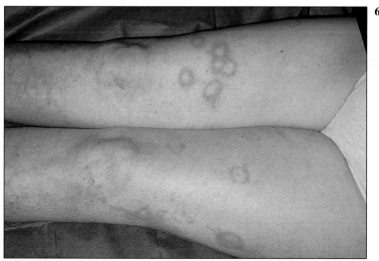

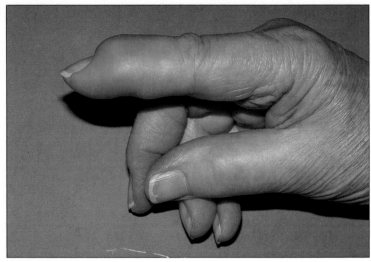

68 This lesion developed overnight in a patient with cardiac failure.
(a) Name the condition.
(b) How can it be confirmed?
(c) What may have caused it?

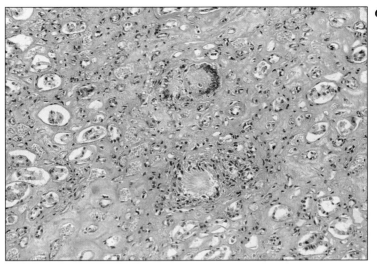

69 This renal biopsy is from a patient with long-standing renal impairment and a history of painful arthropathy. What abnormality is shown?

70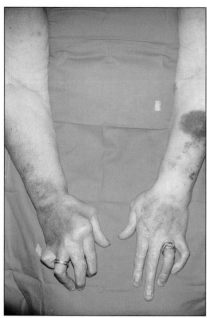

70–73 (a) What abnormal signs are seen in the patient in **70**?
(b) The renal biopsy findings from the same patient are shown in **71–73**. Describe the abnormal features.
(c) What is the diagnosis?

71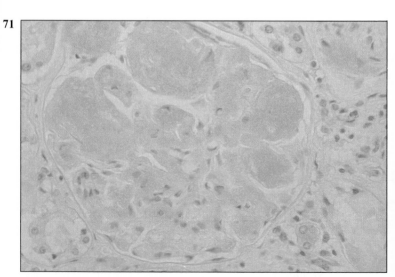

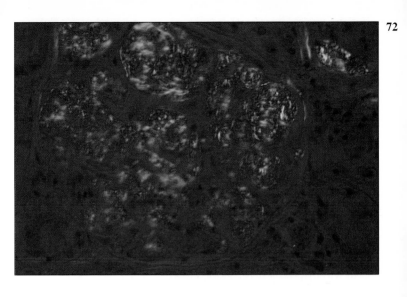

72

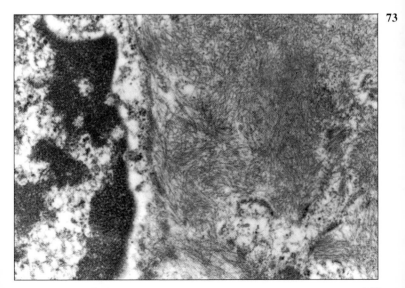

73

74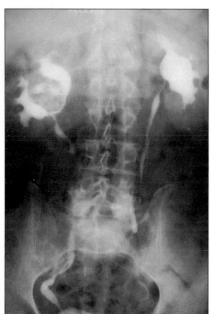

74, 75 What abnormality is noted on the intravenous urogram and in the gross specimen of the kidney?

75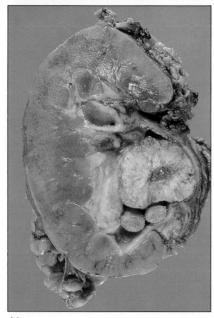

76, 77 What abnormality is shown in the plain abdominal X-ray and in the gross renal specimen?

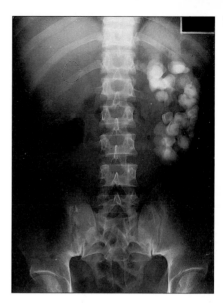

76

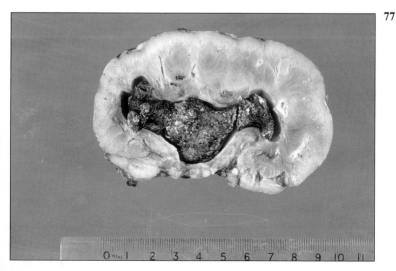

77

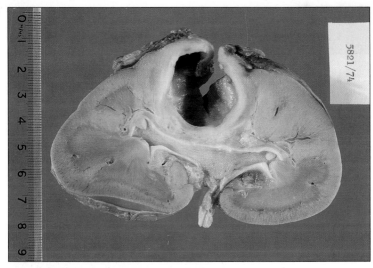

78 The renal specimen is from a patient with painless haematuria and sterile pyuria.
(a) What is the lesion?
(b) What is its likely cause?

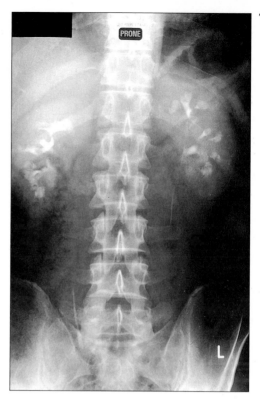

79 (a) What is seen in this intravenous urogram?
(b) What is the likely outcome of this condition?
(c) What are the likely clinical features?

80

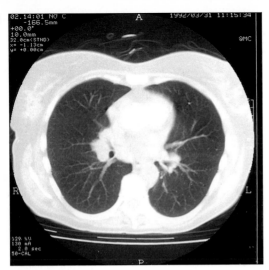

81

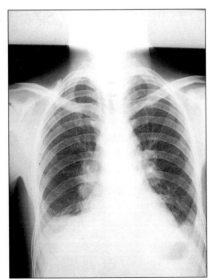

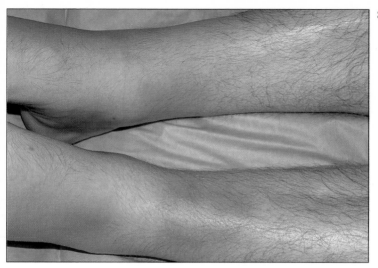

80–82 (a) Name the abnormalities shown on the CT scan and plain X-ray of the chest.
(b) What abnormality is shown in the legs of the patient?
(c) What is the unifying diagnosis?
(d) How may the kidneys be affected in this condition?

83

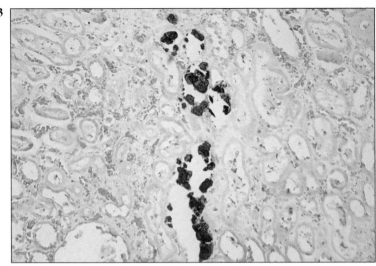

83 What is shown in this renal biopsy stained with Von Kossa stain?

84

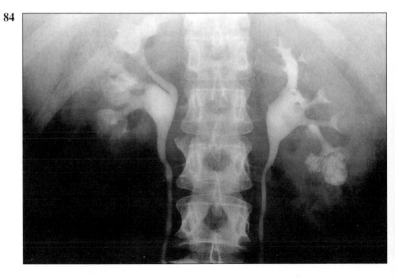

84 What is seen in this intravenous urogram?

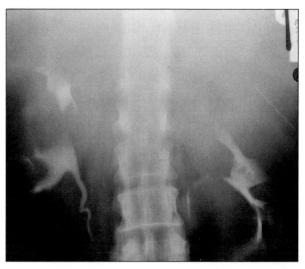

85 What is seen in this intravenous urogram?

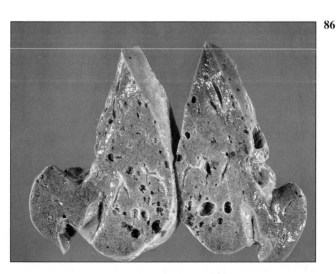

86 (a) What is seen in this pathological specimen?
(b) With which renal condition is it associated?

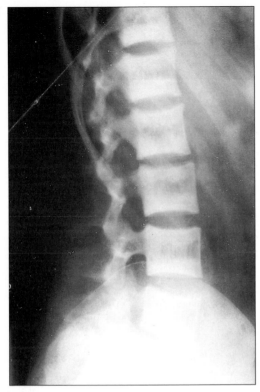

87 What characteristic abnormality is shown on this X-ray from a patient with chronic renal failure?

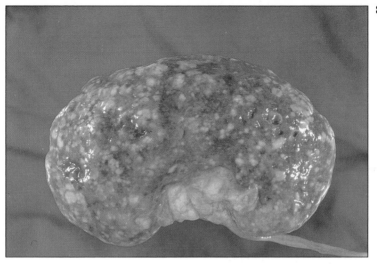

88, 89 The gross specimen is from a patient with a febrile illness and lumbar pain.
(a) What is the diagnosis?
(b) What is shown in the histological specimen?

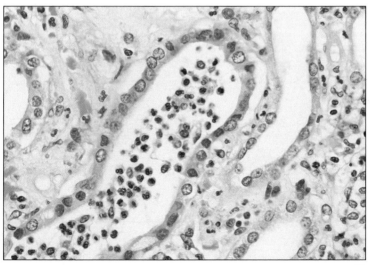

90 What is shown in this intravenous urogram?

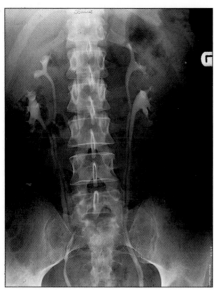

91 What is shown in this blood film from a patient with renal impairment and arthropathy?

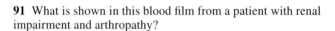

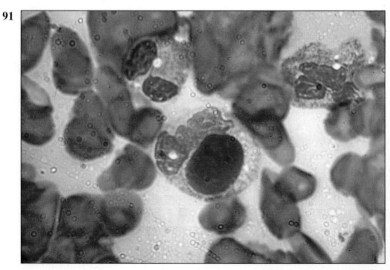

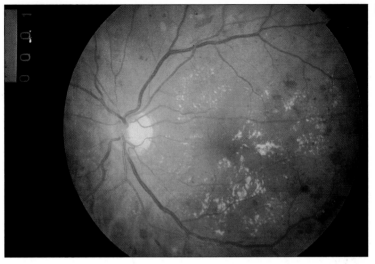

92 (a) What abnormalities are seen?
(b) What is the diagnosis?

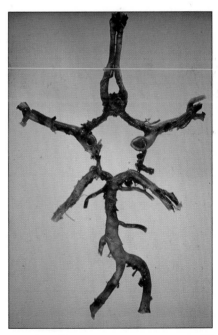

93 (a) What abnormal
feature is seen in this
specimen from a patient
who was on dialysis?
(b) What was the renal
diagnosis?

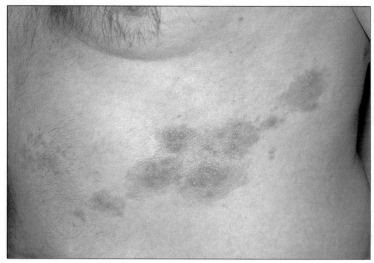

94 This patient has received a renal transplant.
(a) What is the lesion shown?
(b) What is the treatment?

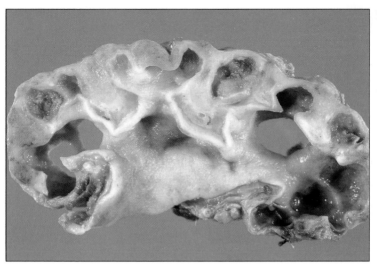

95, 96 The kidney in **95** is from an adult and that in **96** from a child.
(a) What are the renal lesions?
(b) What are the likely causes for each?

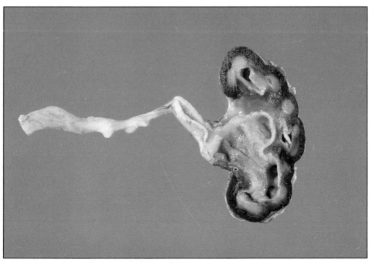

97

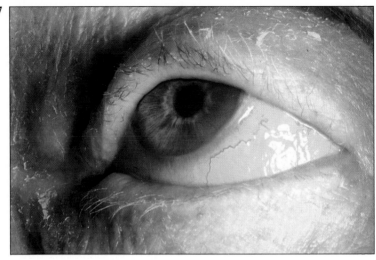

97 What is the sign shown?

98 (a) What is the diagnosis?
(b) How may the kidney be involved in this condition?

98

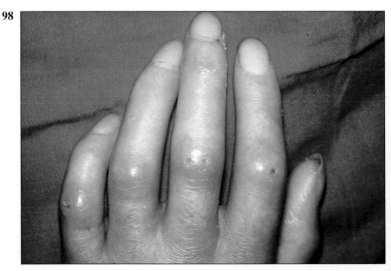

99 (a) What lesion is shown in this patient who has acute renal impairment?
(b) What is the likely diagnosis?

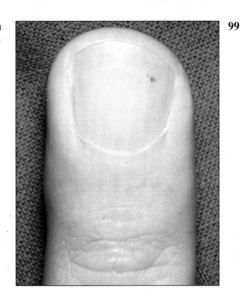

100 This X-ray is from a patient on chronic haemodialysis who complains of a stiff shoulder.
(a) What is seen on X-ray?
(b) What is the cause?

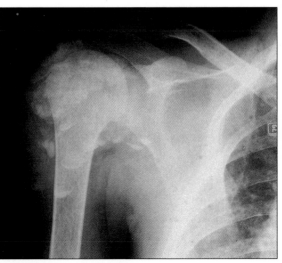

101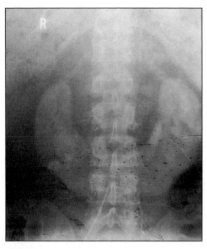

101 (a) What is seen in this illustration?
(b) What clinical features may occur?

102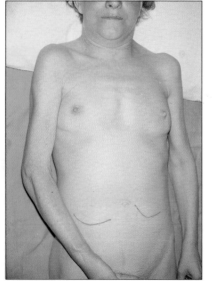

102 (a) Name the signs seen in this patient.
(b) What is the diagnosis?

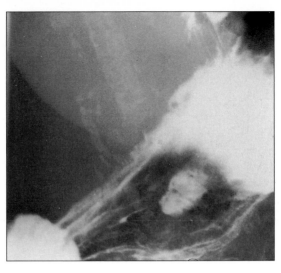

103 A frequent association of chronic renal failure is shown in this illustration. What is the lesion?

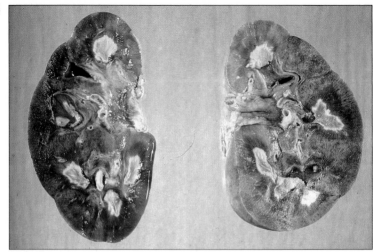

104, 105 (a) What abnormality is seen in the gross specimen of the kidney and on microscopy?
(b) What are the possible causes?

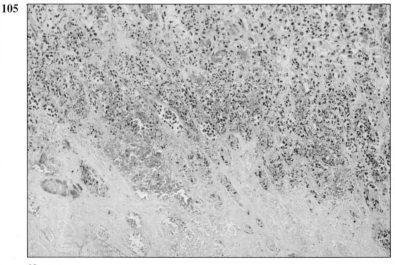

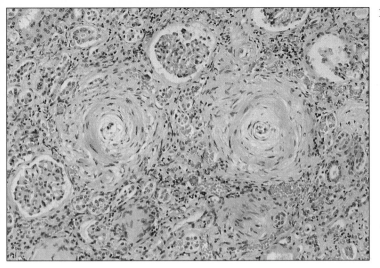

106, 107 These renal biopsy pictures are from a middle-aged lady with long-standing osteoarthritis and renal failure.
(a) What abnormalities are shown?
(b) What is the likely cause?

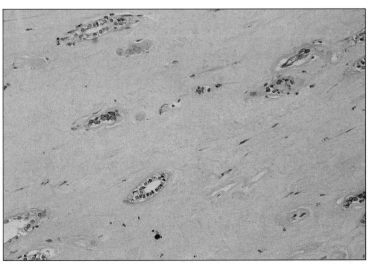

108

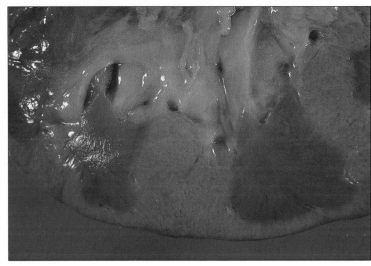

108, 109 (a) What features are shown in the gross specimen and microscopic section?
(b) What is the diagnosis?

109

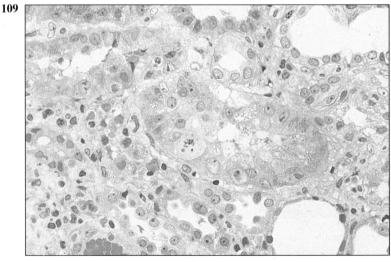

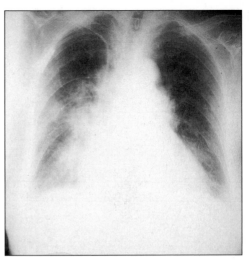

110, 111 These chest radiographs are from the same patient.
(a) What are the abnormalities?
(b) What treatment has the patient received?
(c) What is the likely diagnosis?

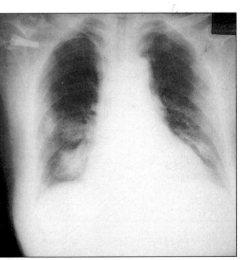

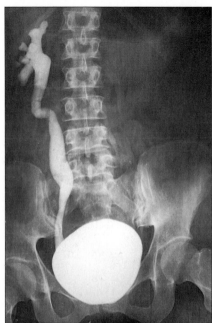

112, 113 What abnormalities are shown in these two micturating cystograms?

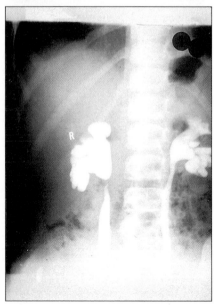

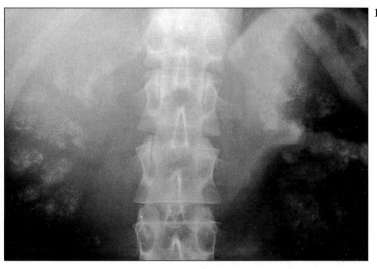

114 What is shown in this plain X-ray of the abdomen?

115 Name the abnormality in this chest radiograph from a patient with chronic renal failure.

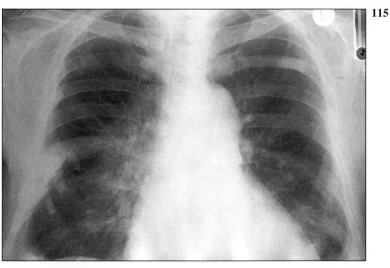

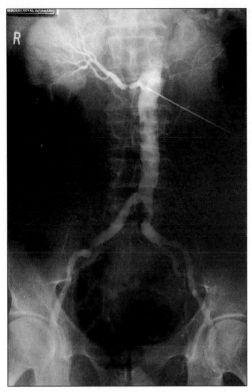

116 (a) Name the investigation.
(b) What abnormal feature is seen?

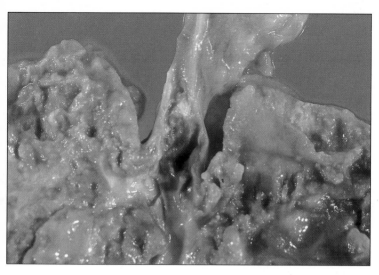

117 What is the abnormality seen at the origin of one of the renal arteries?

118 What sign is shown here?

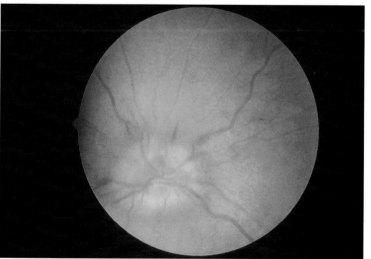

119

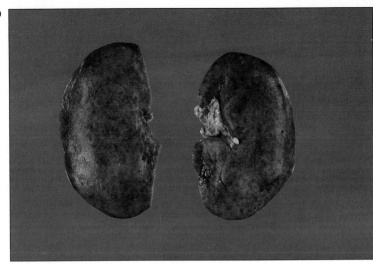

119, 120 These kidneys are from a patient with malignant hypertension. What is seen on histology?

120

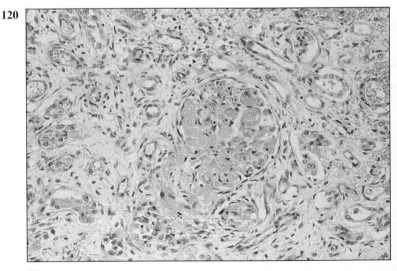

70

121 What is shown in the arteriogram?

121

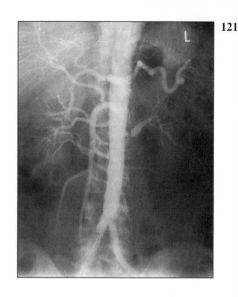

122 This photomicrograph is from a renal biopsy performed on a four-year-old child who developed renal failure following a bout of diarrhoea.
(a) What abnormalities are shown?
(b) What is the likely diagnosis?

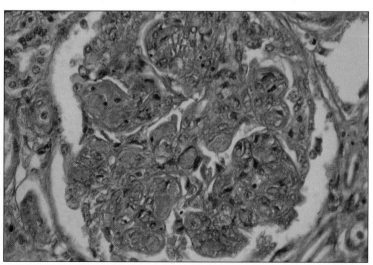

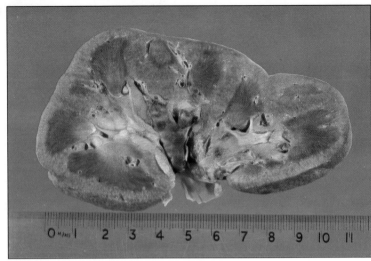

123 This complication developed in a patient with nephrotic syndrome. Name the lesion.

124 These kidneys are from a patient with end-stage renal disease. What was the possible cause of renal failure?

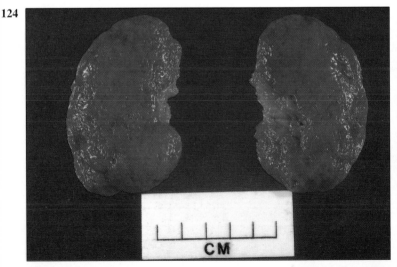

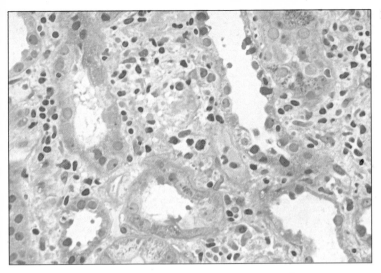

125 This patient suffered an acute deterioration in renal function following treatment with an antibiotic.
(a) What does the light microscopy show?
(b) What was the likely antibiotic?

126 This X-ray is from a patient with renal failure.
(a) What is the diagnosis?
(b) What are the possible reasons for development of renal failure?

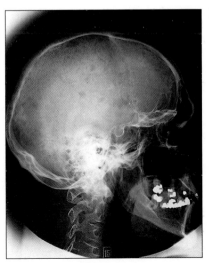

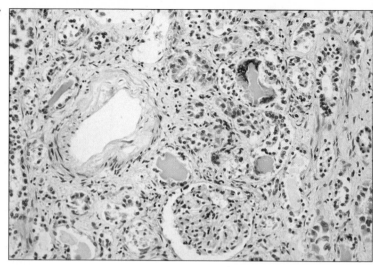

127 What is shown in this renal biopsy from a patient with renal failure and hypercalcaemia?

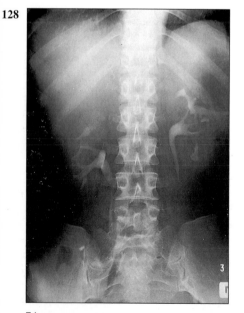

128 This intravenous urogram is from a patient with a hereditary blood disorder.
(a) What is shown?
(b) What is the likely diagnosis?

129 This investigation is from a patient who presented with haematuria.
(a) Name the investigation.
(b) What abnormality is shown?

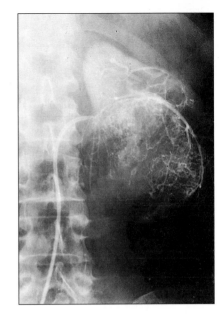

130 What does this specimen show?

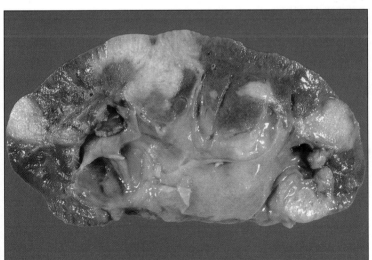

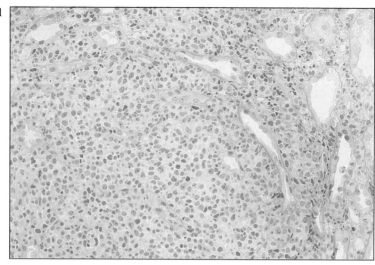

131 This biopsy shows tumour infiltration and is from a patient with renomegaly and haematuria. What is the likely nature of the tumour?

132

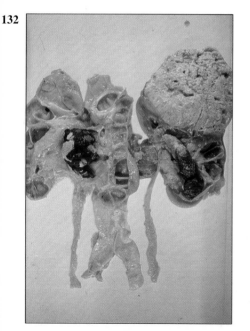

132 Name the two abnormal features in this renal specimen.

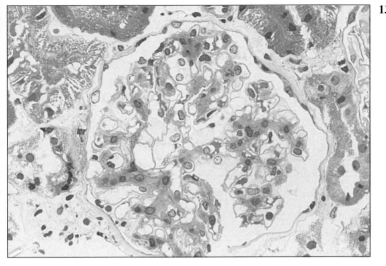

133, 134 What is the obvious abnormal feature in this renal biopsy stained with haematoxylin–eosin and silver?

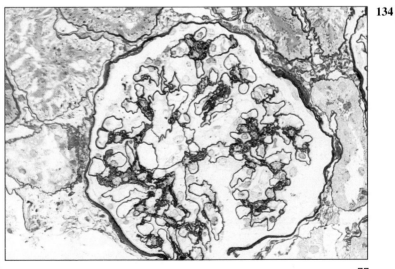

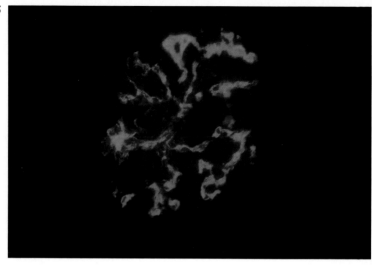

135, 136 These are immunofluorescence and electron micrographs of the preceding biopsy.
(a) What is the likely diagnosis?
(b) What are the modes of presentation of patients with this disorder?

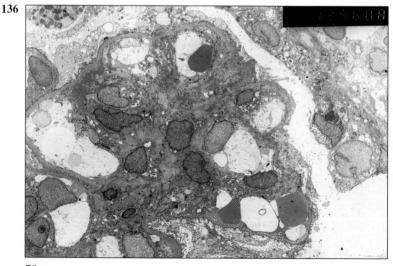

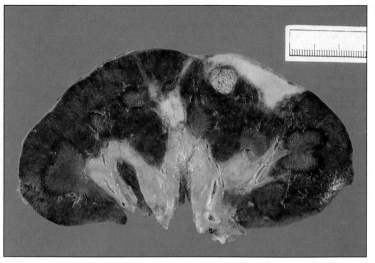

137 This kidney is from a patient who presented with flank pain and haematuria. What is the diagnosis?

138 What is the abnormal feature in this biopsy?

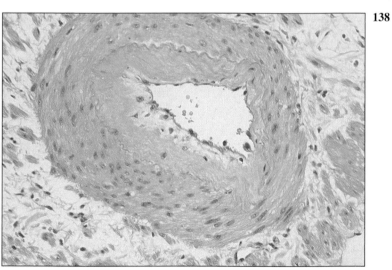

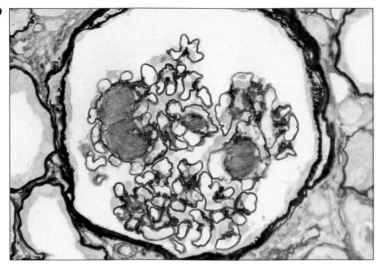

139, 140 (a) What is this lesion?
(b) What caused it?

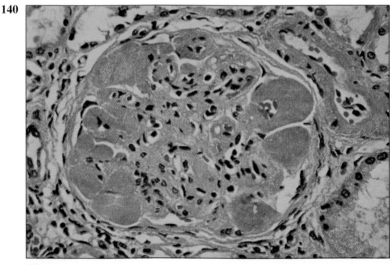

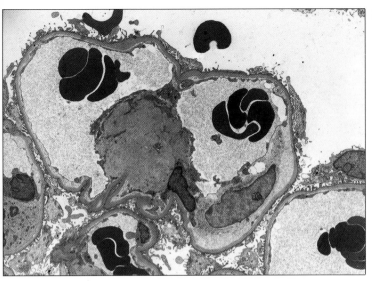

141 What changes of diabetic nephropathy are shown in this electronmicrograph?

142 What complication has occurred in this patient who received a renal transplantation five years previously?

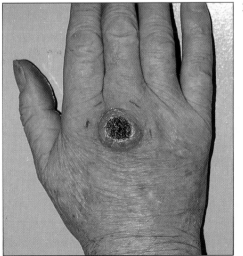

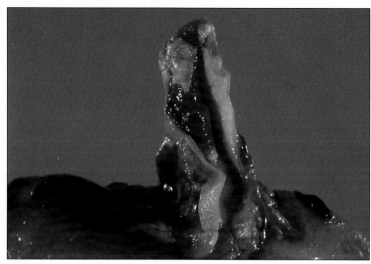

143 What is the pathological diagnosis?

144 What is the pathological diagnosis?

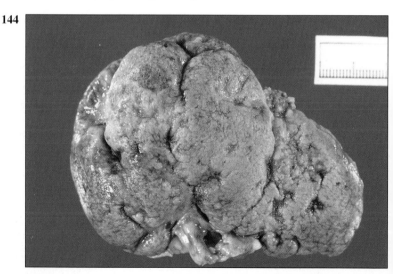

145 What abnormality is
shown in this intravenous
urogram?

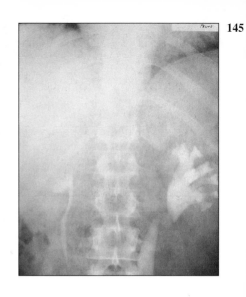

146 Of what is this intravenous urogram diagnostic?

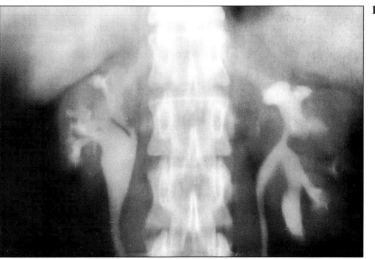

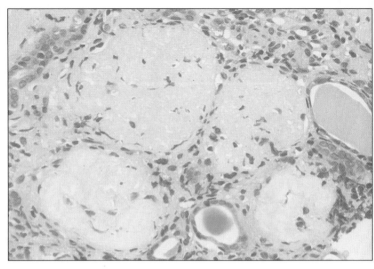

147 (a) Describe this histological picture.
(a) What is the cause?

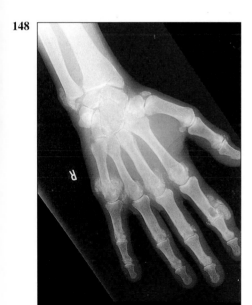

148 This X-ray was taken from a man with chronic renal failure. What does it show?

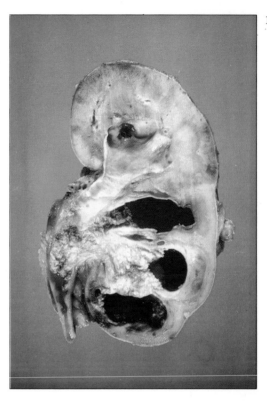

149 What is the diagnosis?

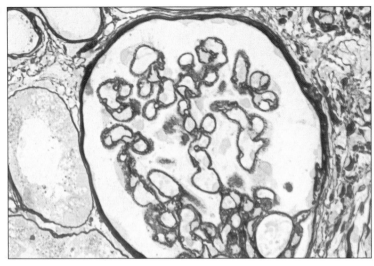

150, 151 These biopsy pictures are from a patient with nephrotic syndrome. (**151** shows immunofluorescence staining for IgG.)
(a) What are the abnormalities?
(b) What is the diagnosis?

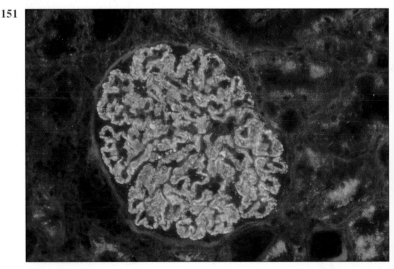

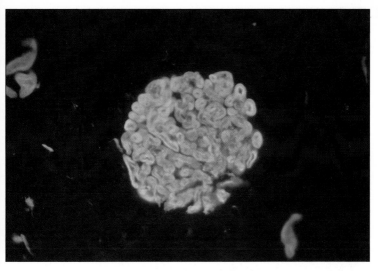

152 This biopsy is from a female who developed a complication of pregnancy. Immunofluorescence was performed with antibodies against fibrinogen. What was the complication?

153 What is the diagnosis in this child with renal failure?

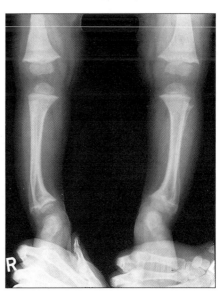

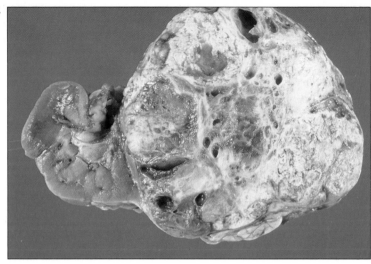

154, 155 Which renal tumour is shown here?

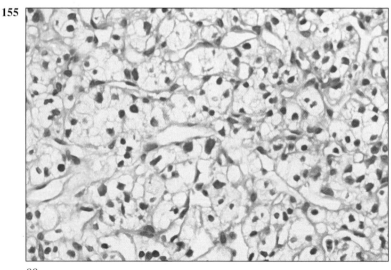

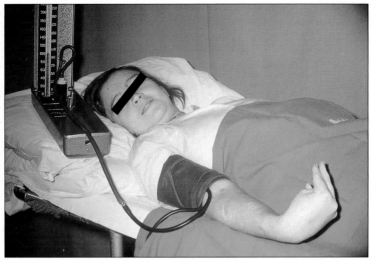

156 (a) What sign is shown in this patient on chronic dialysis?
(b) What type of surgery has she undergone?

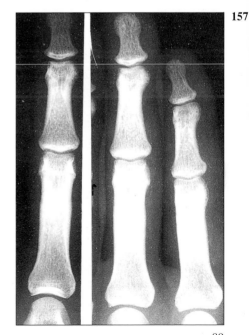

157 (a) What abnormal
radiological feature is
illustrated?
(b) What is the cause?

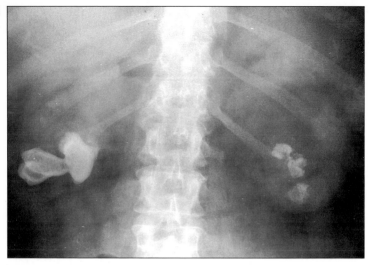

158 What is shown on this plain radiograph of the abdomen?

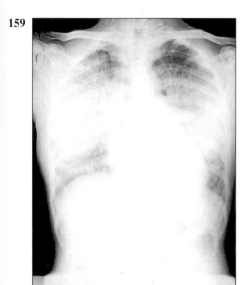

159 What is the diagnosis?

160 (a) What abnormality is shown in this child with chronic renal failure ?
(b) How could it have been prevented?

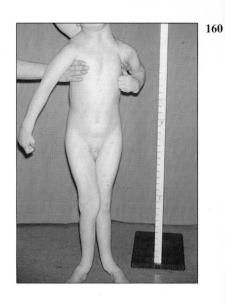

161 (a) What is the diagnosis?
(b) Why?

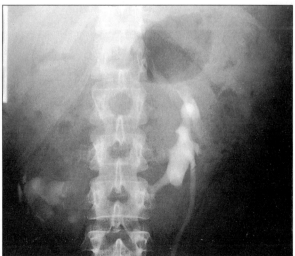

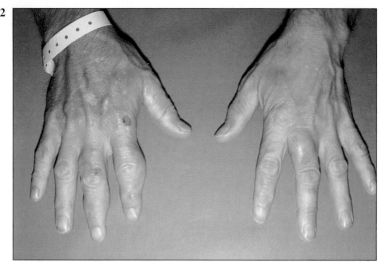

162, 163 What is shown here in a chronic haemodialysis patient?

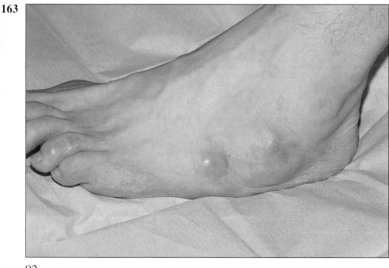

164 (a) What sign
is shown?
(b) What is the
likely cause?

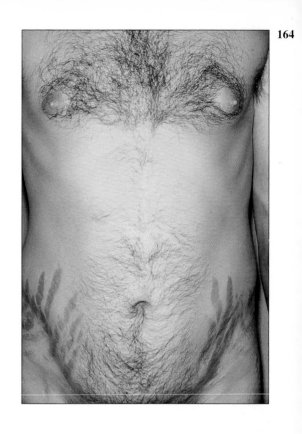

165 What is the
likely diagnosis?

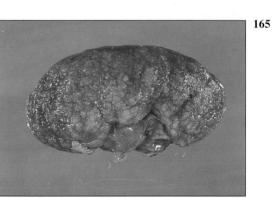

166

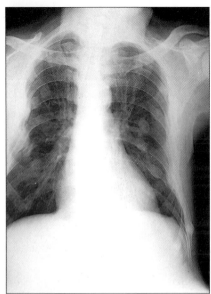

166 What complication of renal bone disease is seen?

167 This patient has been on dialysis for ten years.
(a) What sign is shown?
(b) What procedure has been performed?

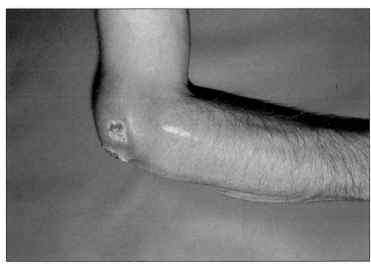

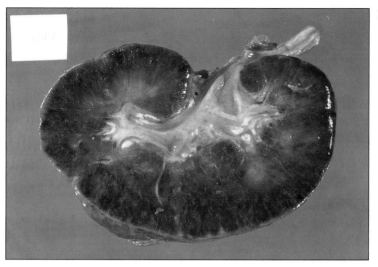

168 This transplanted kidney was removed several weeks after transplantation. What was the diagnosis?

169 (a) What abnormal features are seen in this transplant biopsy? (b) What is the diagnosis and treatment?

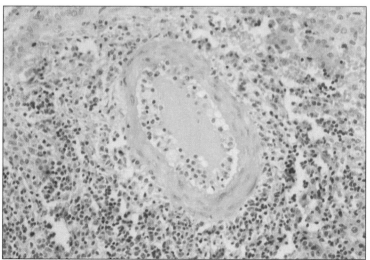

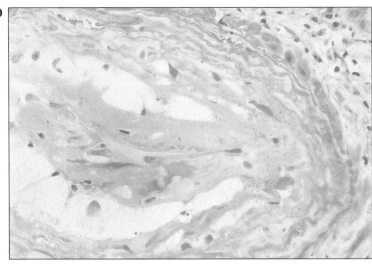

170, 171 This is the renal transplant biopsy of a patient who received the graft five years ago and has a serum creatinine of 250 µmol/l. The picture shows part of an intrarenal artery. What is the diagnosis and treatment?

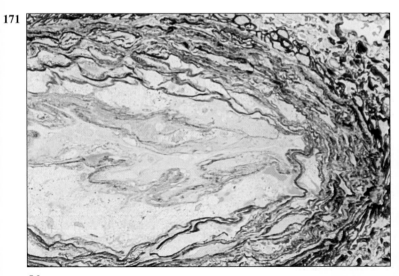

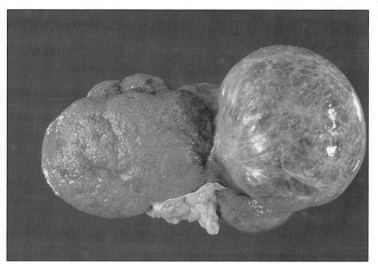

172 What is the pathological diagnosis and clinical presentation?

173 What is the abnormal pathology?

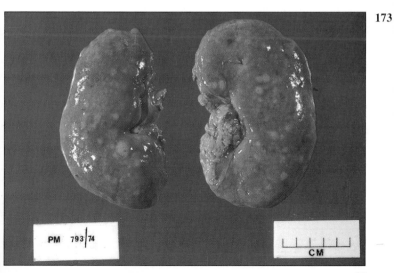

PM 793/74

CM

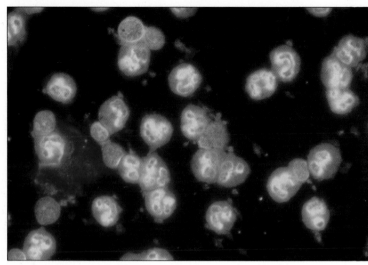

174, 175 (a) What immunological test is illustrated in these photomicrographs?
(b) What is its significance?

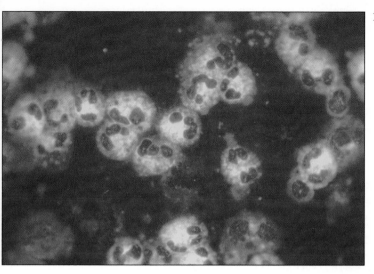

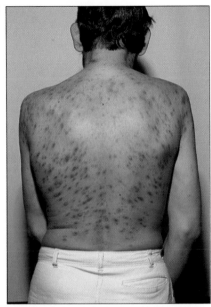

176–178 (a) What is the lesion shown in this patient on chronic dialysis?
(b) What procedure has been performed?
(c) What does the histology show?
(d) How was the lesion treated?

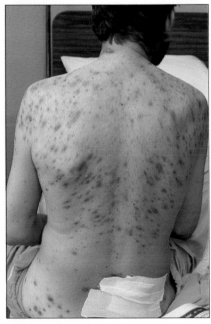

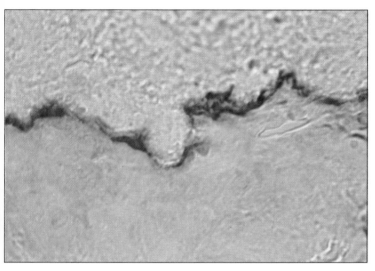

179 These kidneys are from a patient with adenoma sebaceum and a history of seizures. What is the diagnosis?

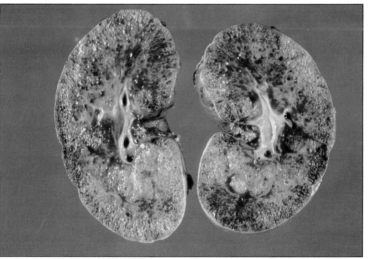

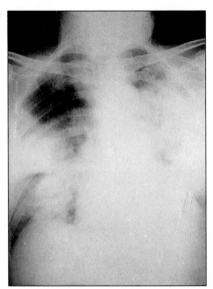

180, 181 What is the diagnosis?

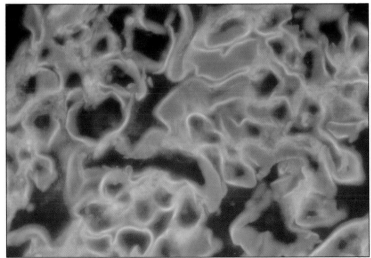

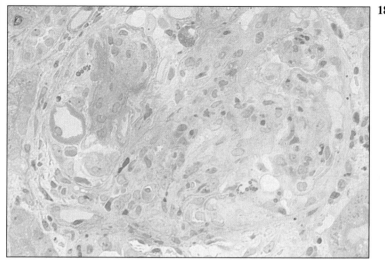

182, 183 This renal biopsy is from a patient with positive antinuclear antibody and renal failure. What is the diagnosis?

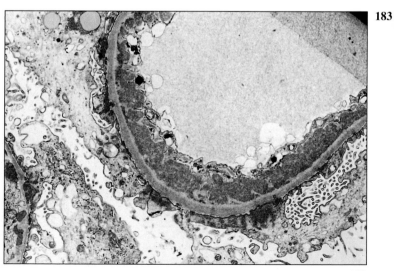

184

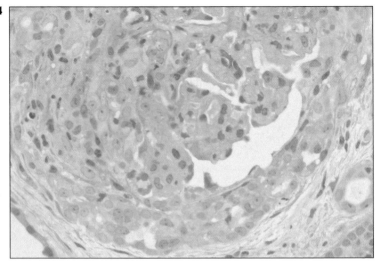

184, 185 What is the abnormality?

185

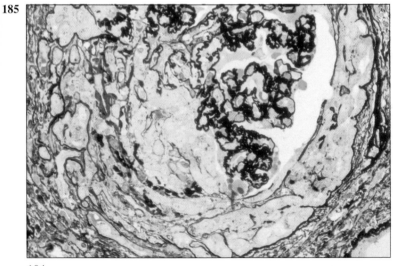

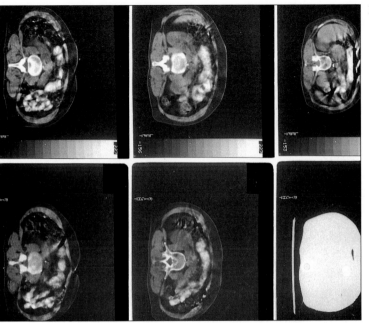

186 What is the finding on this CT scan of abdomen?

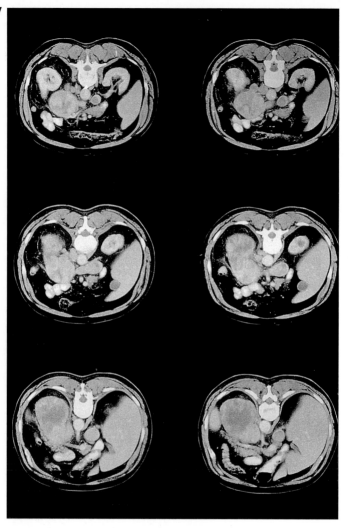

187 What lesion is seen on this CT scan?

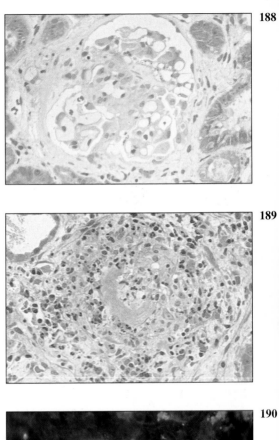

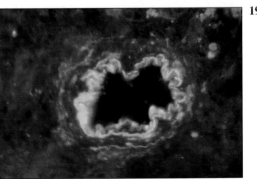

188–190 Describe the features shown in these illustrations of renal biopsy. The immunofluorescence is stained for C3.

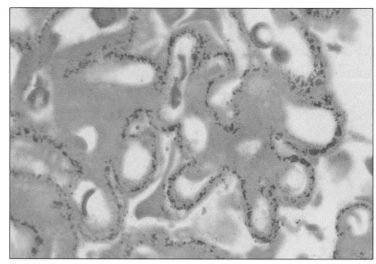

191 Fresh biopsy material was unavailable for immunofluorescence. Immunogold staining for IgG was used on fixed tissue. What is the diagnosis?

192 What is shown in this post mortem histology from a patient who had severe jaundice and renal failure?

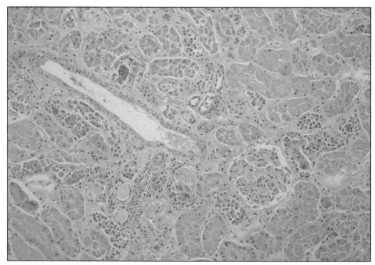

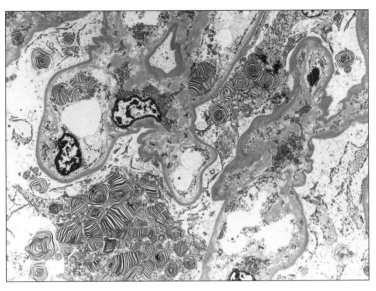

193 This biopsy shows a characteristic glomerular feature of an inherited disorder associated with renal failure.
(a) Name the abnormality and the disorder.
(b) Name three clinical features apart from renal failure.

194 (a) What instrument is illustrated?
(b) What is its use in nephrology?

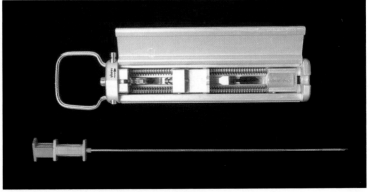

195

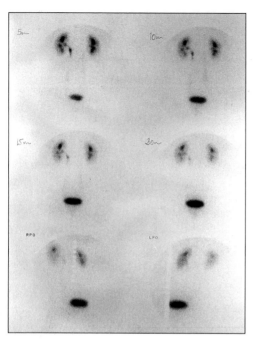

195, 196 What is shown here?

196

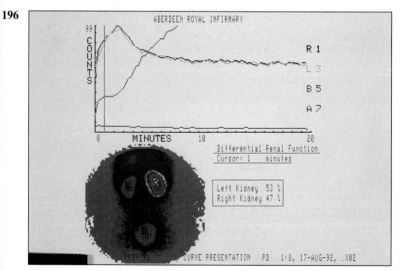

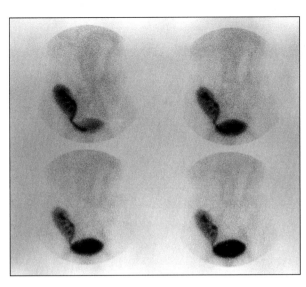

197, 198 What is shown in this isotope renogram?

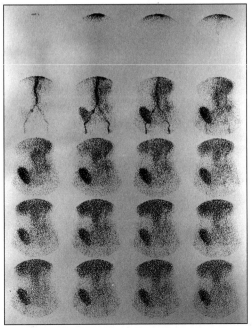

199, 200 (a) What lesion is illustrated?
(b) How has it been treated?

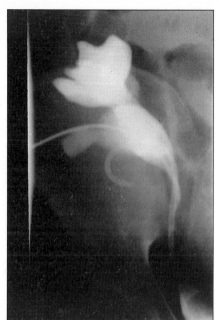

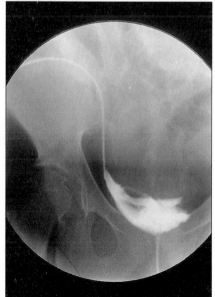

112

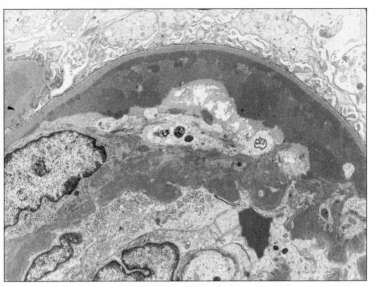

201 This is an electronmicrograph from a patient who presented with the nephrotic syndrome. The picture shows massive glomerular subendothelial dense deposits and mesangial interpositioning. What is the diagnosis?

Answers

1, 2 (a) Thrombosis of the subclavian vein.
(b) Thrombolysis.
(c) Subclavian vein catheterization.

3, 4 Stenosis of the subclavian vein before and after angioplasty.

5 (a) Arteriovenous shunt.
(b) Vascular access for haemodialysis and haemofiltration, especially in patients with clotting disorders.

6 Arteriovenous graft.

7 Acne and (clotted) arteriovenous fistula. Acne is a feature associated with steroids given for immunosuppression

8 Umbilical hernia associated with CAPD (Continuous Ambulatory Peritoneal Dialysis).

9 (a) Pericardial effusion.
(b) Dialysis.
(c) Cardiac tamponade.

10, 11 (a) Left nephrectomy.
(b) Adult polycystic kidney disease.
(c) Nephrectomy may be required in APKD (Autosomal-dominant Polycystic Kidney Disease) for the following reasons: (1) in the case of severe pain due to rupture, haemorrhage or pressure; (2) to create space for renal graft.

12 (a) Half-and-half nails (Moon nails).
(b) Uraemia.

13–15 (a) Livedo reticularis.
(b) Glomerulopathy leading to nephrotic syndrome.
(c) Cryoglobulinaemia.

16 Small pneumothorax on the left side due to catheterization of subclavian vein.

17 Left ectopic pelvic kidney.

18 (a) Vascular calcification.
(b) Result of hyperphosphataemia and hyperparathyroidism leading to elevated calcium phosphate product.

19 (a) Retrograde pyelogram.
(b) Emphysematous pyelonephritis due to gas-forming bacteria.

20 (a) Renal failure associated with rheumatoid arthritis can be due to: (1) analgesic nephropathy; (2) renal amyloidosis; (3) membranous nephropathy secondary to gold or penicillamine (rare).
(b) This patient is receiving dialysis via a subclavian catheter.

21–23 (a) Henoch–Schoenlein purpura.
(b) Glomeruli show proliferation of mesangial cells.

24 (a) Subconjunctival haemorrhage due to thrombocytopenia.
(b) This resulted from azathioprine treatment.

25, 26 (a) Dialysis-associated amyloidosis due to accumulation of β-2 microglobulin.
(b) Surgery for carpal tunnel syndrome.

27 Radio-opaque bladder calculi.

28 (a) Koilonychia.
(b) Iron-deficiency anaemia in patients with renal failure may occur following blood loss from the gut and during haemodialysis.

29 (a) Avascular necrosis of the femoral head following treatment with steroids.
(b) The patient had a renal transplant.

30 (a) Sine waves and peaked T-waves.
(b) Hyperkalaemia.
(c) Treatment is urgent and comprises: (1) intravenous calcium gluconate; (2) insulin and glucose infusion, bicarbonate infusion, nebulized salbutamol; (3) calcium resonium orally or rectally; (4) dialysis.

31 Hypochromia; anisocytosis; burr cells.

32–34 (a) Partial lipodystrophy.
(b) Type-II membranoproliferative glomerulonephritis (dense deposit disease).

35, 36 (a) Adult polycystic disease.
(b) Cyst lined by epithelium.

37, 38 Thin basement membrane state.

39–42 Normal kidney with a normal histological appearance.

43, 44 Scar of parathyroidectomy and pseudoclubbing.

45–49 (a) Oedema and ascites.
(b) **47** shows lipid accumulation in tubules; **48** shows a normal glomerular basement membrane; **49** illustrates loss of foot processes seen in this case of minimal change disease.
(c) Nephrotic syndrome.

50–52 (a) Oedema.
(b) Membranous nephropathy. The spikes in **52** are due to subepithelial deposits in the glomerular basement membrane.

53 Electron-dense deposits. These form subepithelially and are then surrounded by new basement membrane material.

54 Multicystic dysplastic kidney.

55 Double ureter.

56 Urinary tract infection, calculi and urinary obstruction.

57, 58 (a) CAPD catheter *in situ*.
(b) Gas under the diaphragm.
(c) Laparotomy and removal of catheter.

59 Candidiasis in an immunosuppressed patient.

60, 61 Diffuse post-infectious proliferative glomerulonephritis.

62, 63 Focal segmental glomerulosclerosis.

64, 65 (a) Wilms' tumour.
(b) The histology shows sheets of tumour cells.

66, 67 (a) Erythema multiforme (target lesions) and oedema.
(b) Common causes include mycoplasma, streptococcal infections, viral infections and drugs such as sulphonamide.

68 (a) Acute gout.
(b) Aspiration of joint and examination by microscopy for uric acid crystals.
(c) Diuretics are a common cause of acute gout in patients with cardiac failure.

69 Uric acid crystals. This patient suffers from gouty nephropathy.

70–73 (a) Purpura and echymoses of the skin and hand deformities characteristic of rheumatoid arthritis.
(b) **71** is a Congo red stain showing amorphous material in glomerulus. **72** shows the apple-green birefringence and **73** shows the appearance of fibrillary material on electron microscopy.
(c) The diagnosis is renal amyloidosis secondary to rheumatoid arthritis.

74, 75 The intravenous urogram shows filling defects in a dilated right renal pelvis. The kidney shows a pelvic transitional cell carcinoma and stones.

76, 77 The plain X-ray shows a staghorn calculus in the left kidney. The gross specimen reveals a large staghorn calculus.

78 (a) Renal abscess.
(b) Tuberculosis.

79 (a) Tubular ectasia characteristic of medullary sponge kidneys.
(b) The usual course is benign.
(c) Patients may develop renal calculi, renal tubular acidosis and bacteruria.

80–82 (a) The CT scan and chest X-ray show bilateral hilar adenopathy.
(b) The legs show erythema nodosum.
(c) Sarcoidosis is the likely diagnosis.
(d) Nephrolithiasis, hypercalcaemia, nephrocalcinosis and, rarely, glomerulopathy and sarcoid granulomatous interstitial nephropathy may occur in sarcoidosis.

83 Nephrocalcinosis.

84 Stone in the left lower pole of the kidney.

85 Polycystic kidneys.

86 (a) Hepatic cysts.
(b) These are seen in about one-third of patients with autosomal dominant polycystic kidney disease.

87 Rugger-jersey spine appearance in renal osteodystrophy.

88, 89 (a) Acute pyelonephritis.
(b) Acute inflammatory cell infiltrate in the tubule.

90 Bilateral duplex kidneys.

91 Lupus erythematosis cells. These are neutrophils with ingested lymphocyte nuclei seen in patients with systemic lupus erythematosis.

92 (a) Dot haemorrhages and hard exudates.
(b) Background diabetic retinopathy.

93 (a) Anterior communicating artery aneurysm.
(b) Autosomal dominant polycystic disease.

94 (a) Herpes zoster (shingles).
(b) Acyclovir.

95, 96 (a) Hydronephrotic kidneys.
(b) In adults it is commonly due to strictures, calculi, prostatic enlargement, tumours of the urinary tract and pelvic tumours. In children vesico-ureteric reflux, ureteric strictures and congenital deformities such as posterior urethral valves are likely causes.

97 Band keratopathy seen in hyperparathyroidism.

98 (a) Scleroderma.
(b) Uraemia associated with malignant hypertension (scleroderma crisis) may occur.

99 (a) Splinter haemorrhage.
(b) Subacute bacterial endocarditis associated with acute glomerulo-nephritis.

100 (a) Calcification of periarticular soft-tissue.
(b) Increased calcium phosphate product as a result of secondary hyperparathyroidism and hyperphosphataemia.

101 (a) Nephrogram of horseshoe kidney.
(b) Calculi, ureteric obstruction and urinary tract infection.

102 (a) Uremic pallor, arteriovenous fistula in right arm, bilateral loin swelling.
(b) Autosomal dominant polycystic disease.

103 Barium-filled crater of a gastric ulcer.

104, 105 (a) Renal papillary necrosis.
(b) Analgesic nephropathy; diabetes mellitus; sickle-cell disease; acute pyelonephritis.

106, 107 (a) Tubular atrophy, medullary fibrosis, interstitial inflammation and intimal thickening.
(b) Analgesic nephropathy.

108, 109 (a) Swelling and pallor of the cortex. A mitotic figure can be seen in a tubular cell.
(b) Acute tubular necrosis.

110, 111 (a) Pulmonary opacities, pulmonary oedema and cardiomegaly.
(b) The patient has received haemodialysis and ultrafiltration via the right subclavian catheter.
(c) Wegener's granulomatosis.

112, 113 Grade-3 unilateral and bilateral vesico-ureteric reflux.

114 Nephrocalcinosis in medullary sponge kidney.

115 Heterotopic calcification.

116 (a) Lumbar aortogram.
(b) Stenosis of the left renal artery.

117 Stenosis of renal artery due to atheroma.

118 Papilloedema.

119, 120 Fibrinoid necrosis of the glomerular afferent arteriole and of a portion of the glomerulus.

121 Stenosis of the left renal artery and poststenotic dilatation.

122 (a) Microthrombi in glomerular capillaries.
(b) Haemolytic uraemic syndrome.

123 Thrombosis of the renal vein.

124 Chronic glomerulonephritis. Small granular kidneys (nephrosclerosis).

125 (a) Acute interstitial nephritis.
(b) Methicillin.

126 (a) Osteolytic lesions of multiple myeloma.
(b) Hypercalcaemia, amyloidosis and myeloma kidney can cause renal failure.

127 Myeloma kidney showing paraprotein casts and associated giant cells.

128 (a) Renal papillary necrosis.
(b) Sickle-cell anaemia.

129 (a) Renal arteriogram.
(b) Tumour vascularity.

130 Metastatic carcinoma in the kidney.

131 Lymphoma.

132 Renal tumour and calculi.

133, 134 Prominent proliferation of mesangial cells and matrix accumulation.

135, 136 (a) IgA disease. The immunofluorescence sample shows IgA and the electron micrograph shows proliferation of mesangial cells and immune complex deposits.
(b) Patients may present with haematuria (gross or microscopic), proteinuria, hypertension and renal impairment. Rarely presenting features include nephrotic syndrome and rapidly progressive renal failure.

137 Renal infarction.

138 Hypertensive arteriosclerosis.

139, 140 (a) Nodular glomerulosclerosis.
(b) Diabetes mellitus.

141 Nodular mesangial sclerosis.

142 Skin cancer. Both squamous and basal cell carcinomas are frequent complications of long-term immunosuppression following renal transplantation.

143 Thrombosis of the renal artery.

144 Chronic pyelonephritis.

145 Hydro-ureteronephrosis.

146 Chronic pyelonephritis showing distortion of the calyces.

147 (a) End-stage hyalinized glomeruli.
(b) These characterize end-stage glomerular renal disease from any cause.

148 Calcification of soft tissue.

149 Transitional cell carcinoma of the renal pelvis associated with hydronephrosis.

150, 151 (a) The light microscopy shows thickening of the basement membrane and 'spikes' of new basement membrane material on the outer aspect of the basement membrane. The immunofluorescence sample in **151** stained with IgG shows granular deposits along glomerular capillary walls.
(b) These are characteristic features of membranous glomerulonephritis.

152 Eclampsia of pregnancy.

153 Renal rickets.

154, 155 Renal cell carcinoma.

156 (a) Chvostek's sign due to hypocalcaemia.
(b) Parathyroidectomy.

157 (a) Subperiosteal bone erosion.
(b) Hyperparathyroidism.

158 Bilateral renal calculi.

159 Bat's wing pulmonary oedema.

160 (a) Renal rickets.
(b) Administration of 1-α hydroxycholicalciferol or calcitriol and control of hyperphosphataemia may have prevented this condition.

161 (a) This intravenous urogram shows a horseshoe kidney.
(b) The clue to diagnosis is that the renal pelvis is facing medially.

162, 163 Metastatic calcification of soft tissue.

164 (a) Abdominal striae.
(b) Treatment with steroids.

165 Granular kidney of a hypertensive patient.

166 Healed multiple rib fractures.

167 (a) Metastatic calcification.
(b) Parathyroid implantation in elbow.

168 Acute rejection.

169 (a) Infiltration of renal vessel by lymphocytes.
(b) Acute vascular rejection. Treatment is with high-dose steroids, antilymphocyte globulin and specific monoclonal antibodies against T-cell receptor CD3 (OK T3).

170, 171 Chronic vascular rejection. There is no specific treatment for this disorder.

172 Simple renal cyst. This is almost always asymptomatic.

173 Tumour deposits (leukaemic). Acute pyelonephritis would enter into the differential diagnosis.

174, 175 (a) Indirect immunofluorescence showing positive antineutrophil cytoplasmic antibody (ANCA) tests: perinuclear ANCA (**174**) and cytoplasmic ANCA (**175**).
(b) This test is highly sensitive but not specific for Wegener's granulomatosis and microscopic polyarteritis.

176–178 (a) Prurigo nodularis.
(b) Bone biopsy from the iliac crest was performed before treatment.
(c) Microscopy of bone shows aluminium in osteoid.
(d) The lesion was treated with desferrioxamine.

179 Cystic kidneys associated with tuberous sclerosis.

180, 181 Goodpasture's syndrome. The immunofluorescence sample shows linear deposit of anti-GBM antibody of IgG class.

182, 183 Systemic lupus erythematosis. The light microscopy and electron microscopy show wire loop lesion.

184, 185 Crescentic glomerulonephritis on haematoxylin–eosin and silver stain.

186 Horseshoe kidney.

187 Left renal tumour infiltrating renal vein and inferior vena cava.

188–190 Focal proliferative changes in glomeruli, vasculitis in small artery. The immunofluorescence sample shows renal arteriole stained for C3 in vasculitis. These features can be seen in Wegener's granulomatosis.and microscopic polyarteritis.

191 Subepithelial deposits in membranous glomerulonephritis.

192 Bilirubin casts associated with acute tubular necrosis.

193 (a) Zebra-stripe storage bodies. These are seen in Anderson–Fabry's disease (a lipid storage disease). The disorder is due to a deficiency of the enzyme α-galactosidase A.
(b) Clinical features include ataxia, peripheral neuropathy, skin lesion and cardiac failure.

194 (a) Biopty gun with Trucut biopsy needle.
(b) Renal biopsy.

195, 196 Isotope renogram (DTPA scan) of normal kidneys.

197, 198 Transplanted kidney functioning normally.

199, 200 (a) Ureteric obstruction in a transplanted kidney.
(b) It has been treated with the insertion of a percutaneous antegrade stent.

201 Type-I membranoproliferative glomerulonephritis.

Index

Figures refer to the illustration/question/answer number, not the page number.